Work From Home Ergonomics 101

Tips to Improve Your Comfort, Productivity, and Safety While Working Remotely

Morgan Sutherland, L.M.T., C.E.A.S.

Work From Home Ergonomics 101

Tips to Improve Your Comfort, Productivity, and Safety While Working Remotely

Copyright © 2021 Morgan Sutherland, L.M.T., C.E.A.S.

Contents

Medical Disclaimer

The information provided in this book is not intended to be a substitute for professional medical advice, diagnosis, or treatment. Never disregard or delay seeking professional medical advice because of something you read in this book. Never rely on information in this book in place of seeking professional medical advice.

Morgan Sutherland is not responsible or liable for any advice, course of treatment, diagnosis, other information, services, and products you obtain in this book. If you're experiencing any pain or discomfort, please consult your doctor or healthcare provider about whether the exercises mentioned in this book are appropriate for you.

Personal Disclaimer

I am not a doctor. The information I provide is based on my personal experiences and research as a licensed massage therapist. Any recommendations I make about posture, exercise, stretching, and massage should be discussed between you and your professional healthcare provider to prevent any risk to your health.

<u>FREE</u> Work From Home Ergonomics 101 Webinar

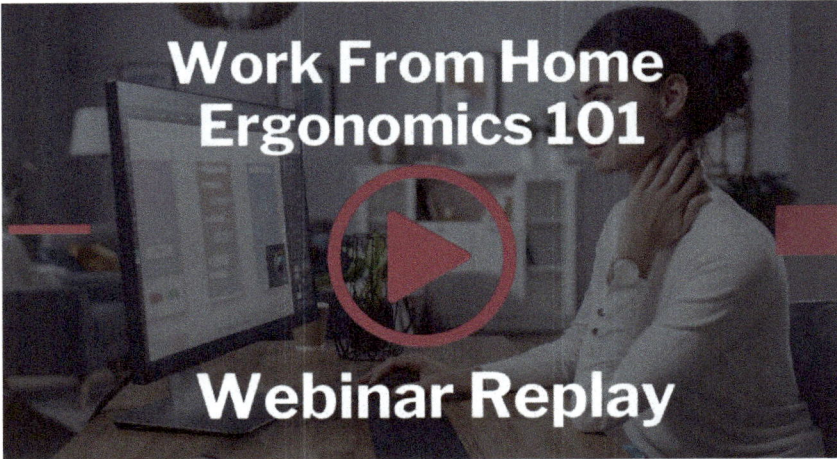

Here's What You'll Learn

- Best practices for safely setting up your home office workstation for optimal comfort and greater productivity.
- How to avoid the four common ergonomic risk factors for injuries by improving your neutral working posture.
- Effective ways to destress at your desk and prevent burnout using breathwork, self-massage, and stretches.

To watch the replay, visit

https://fitergonomics.com/webinar-replay

Introduction

Working remotely from home has many advantages, like cutting your commute time by 100 percent, saving money on gasoline, fewer distractions, and rocking cozy pajamas in the daytime.

Having the flexibility of working in your loungewear while sipping a mocha latte might feel like a godsend. Still, don't ignore the red flags of muscle fatigue caused by awkward postures and a subpar home office setup.

In this book, you will learn the following.

- Practical ergonomic solutions for working from home to improve your comfort, increase productivity, and keep you safe from getting injured.
- Common ergonomic risk factors that can lead to musculoskeletal injuries.
- Warning signs and symptoms of an injury.
- The importance of neutral postures while working from home.
- Best practices for setting up your home office workstation.

- Three microbreaks that can help you recharge so you can prevent burnout.
- How to destress at your desk using breathwork, self-massage, and stretches.
- Valuable tips for troubleshooting everyday aches and pains while working from home.

Injury Is Inevitable Working from Home

Since the coronavirus disease 2019 (COVID-19) pandemic, there seems to be a growing trend of companies embracing the new hybrid work-from-home model. In many cases, employees find themselves working even harder than before to justify not being physically present at work, which can leave them feeling tired, used up, and drained by the end of the workday. And parents who work from home have the added pressure of juggling their work schedules amid the distraction of childcare.

While some companies provide work-from-home stipends, many employees don't have the same setup at home that they had at work. Research has shown that about 72 percent of workers don't have a dedicated office space at home and over half of them aren't working from a dedicated desk for work.

Now, without having a correctly setup workstation and neutral working postures, the chance of getting an injury is just a matter of time. This is why it's essential to understand basic ergonomic principles while working from home so workers can be more comfortable and productive without getting hurt.

What Is Ergonomics?

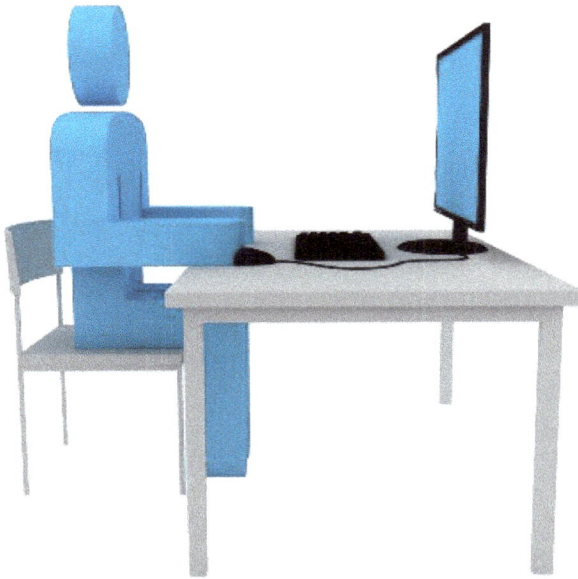

Ergonomics is the science of fitting the jobs to the workers. This includes the equipment and furniture they use and the tasks they need to complete.

In the reverse scenario, when the person is fit to the job, awkward, forceful postures can result in a work-related injury.

Simply put, when conducting an ergonomics assessment, the assessor evaluates the workstation, always with the user in mind. And by doing so, the assessor helps maximize the employee's productivity and performance while reducing discomfort, fatigue, and injury.

Ergonomic Risk Factors

There are four main risk factors to be aware of while working from home: posture, repetition, force, and contact stress. They are all dependent on the frequency and duration of exposure to that risk.

The combination of risk factors can amplify the likelihood of injury. For instance, occasionally working in an awkward posture or for short durations without a lot of repetition or force is unlikely to cause or contribute to a musculoskeletal injury (MSI).

However, combined factors, especially at extreme levels, will always be inherently riskier than any individual risk factor by itself.

Repeated, prolonged, and awkward mid-to-high level exertions are much more common than one-off events and contribute to more MSI development in the office or home office environment.

When home workers can identify these risk factors early enough, they can prevent the onset of a work-related injury.

Awkward Posture

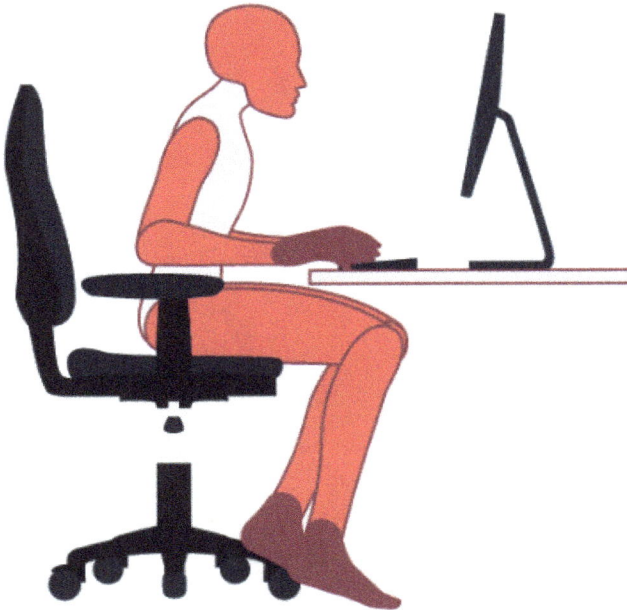

The first risk factor is posture: awkward posture.
Awkward postures are when a person maintains an
unsupported static posture or non-neutral posture
for two hours or more.

Awkward postures, like bending, reaching, and
twisting, can fatigue muscles and slow the blood

flow, so workers might begin to feel tired. This can easily create more opportunities for errors and decrease efficiency, productivity, and accuracy.

Does She Have Neutral Posture?

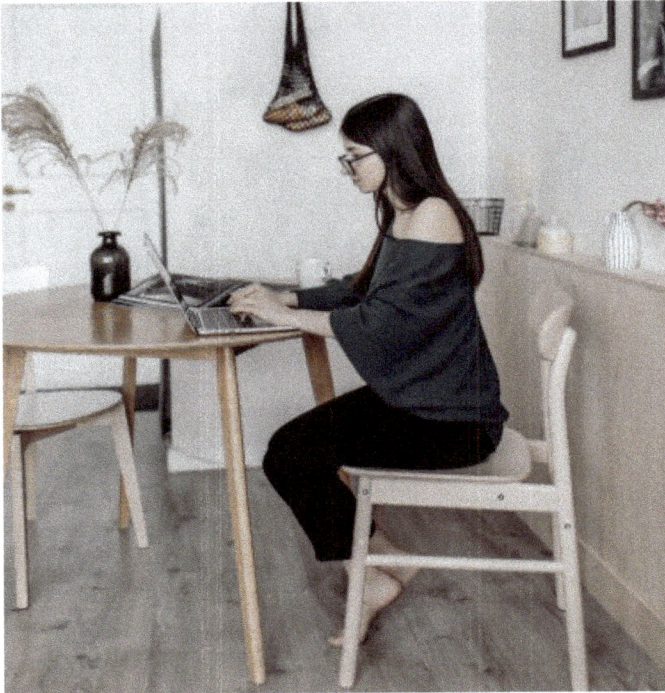

So many of us can relate to this picture of a woman working at the kitchen table, and it might look completely normal. So you might ask, "What's wrong with that?"

Well, let's look at her strengths. Her back is fairly straight, she has good lighting, the room decor is peaceful, and she's not wearing socks. So either the sock fairy stole them out of her laundry basket, or she has control over her thermostat.

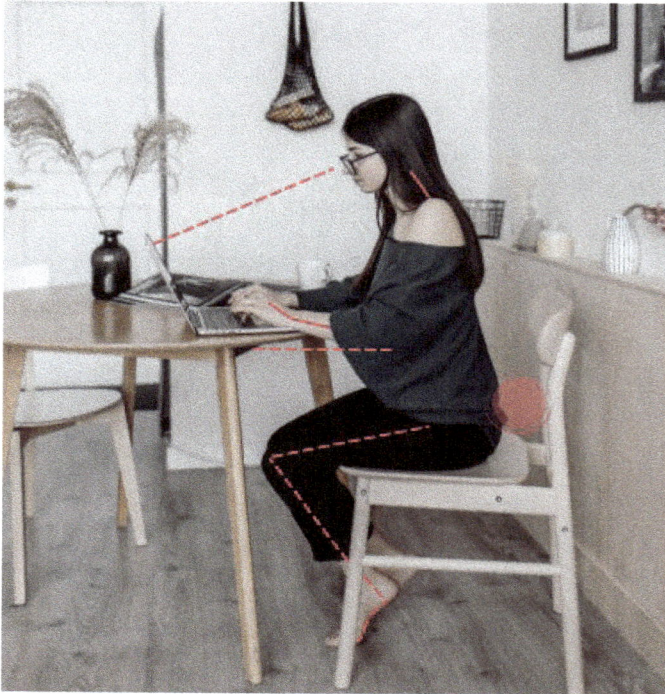

Now, let's look at some opportunities for improvement. The first thing that stands out is that her table height is a little too high for her, and she has to perch forward in her chair to use her laptop, leaving her lower back unsupported.

Because she's using a laptop computer, she has to tilt her head down to view the screen. And to type, she has to hunch her shoulders and then lean into that hard table edge and extend her wrists upward.

And lastly, her feet are pointing down and not flat on the floor.

So this awkward or non-neutral sitting posture might be comfortable for an hour or so, but beyond that, it becomes a risk factor for numerous ergonomic injuries, such as neck strain, carpal tunnel, and low back pain.

.

Repetition

The second risk factor is repetition. When you perform the same task repeatedly, it doesn't give your muscles and tendons enough time to recover. One example is typing for two hours or more without breaks.

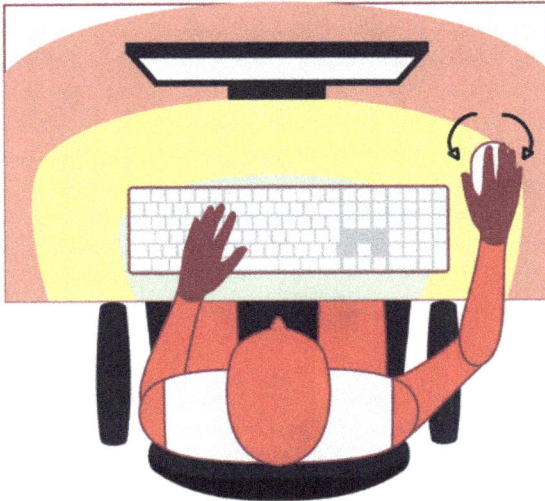

Repetition, when combined with awkward postures, can be the perfect catalyst for an injury. If your workstation is set up so that you need to reach for your mouse repeatedly, don't be surprised if you start to experience stiffness and soreness in your shoulder.

Similar repetitions can occur when using a mouse, and the work hazard might be even more significant because the motions only involve a few fingers on one hand.

Force

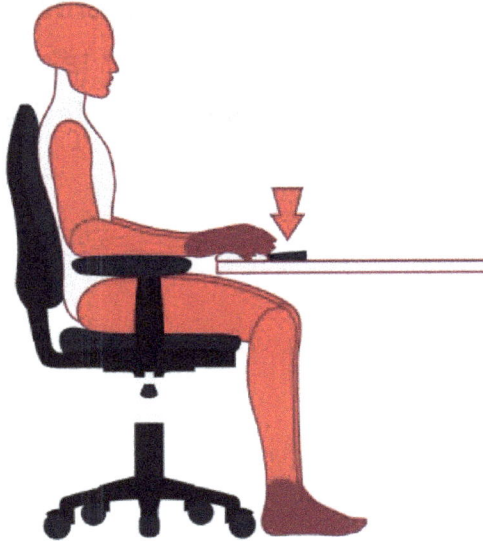

The third risk factor is force. When you're dealing with high-pressure work deadlines, you can find yourself gripping your mouse harder than you're aware of or even typing faster with more force.

Frequent and awkward mouse clicking with a firm grip or keyboard key pounding for prolonged periods (greater than two hours) is more common and risky. This is because force generation with limited recovery time leads to fatigue and reduced circulation.

If it works for you, consider getting a compact keyboard[1] with smaller or flatter keys if you're finding that it requires too much force for you to type. Or you might even consider taking a break from typing and using voice-activated software, like text to speech.

[1] Search online or at a reputable store for compact keyboard, small wireless keyboard, or mini keyboard.

Contact Stress

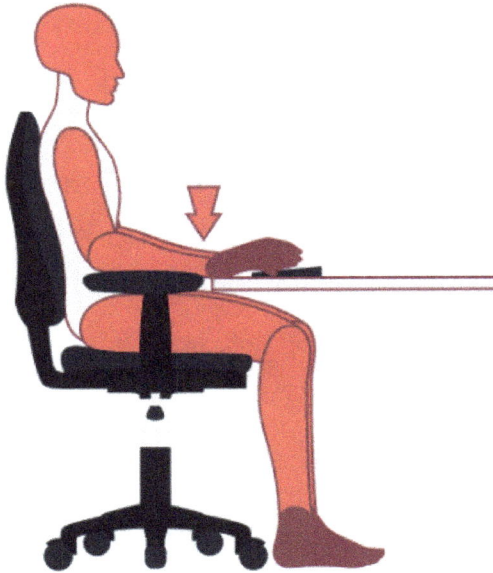

The fourth risk factor is contact stress. Contact stress is when you have continuous pressure for two hours or more against the wrist rest, work surface edge, or armrest with your wrists, forearms, or elbows.

When your muscle tissues get compressed, the underlying ulnar nerve that starts in the neck and passes through the shoulder into the hand also gets compressed, leading to numbness, tingling, pain, and even muscle weakness.

A few do-it-yourself solutions are to cushion the hard table or desk edge with a half-inch to an inch of foam pipe insulation tube, sliced in half horizontally. You could pick that up at your local hardware store—about a $2 option. Or you could go to a website like AliMed.com and purchase a vinyl foam edge protector, which is about $35.

Risk Factor Takeaways

So the big takeaway about risk factors is that you want to ask yourself, "Has my risk changed in my new working environment?"

You need to become more mindful of your posture and your safety. Think about how often and how long you might be exposing yourself to any of these risk factors, so you don't end up getting an injury.

Warning Signs and Symptoms

So now that you know the risk factors, the next step is to recognize warning signs and symptoms of an injury, as they can indicate a potential for an ergonomic risk at your workstation.

Some **common warning signs** that indicate ergonomic risk are redness or swelling around the affected joint, the skin around the area being warm to the touch, and a reduced range of motion for that affected joint.

Some **warning symptoms** that you might encounter include the following.

- fatigue
- soreness
- achiness
- burning
- clumsiness
- stiffness
- tenderness
- tingling
- numbness
- weakness
- change of skin color

When you're exposed to any of these ergonomic risk factors repeatedly or for long periods, and you don't address any of the warning signs and symptoms, you might experience pain or discomfort.

That said, I have you covered because, in the following pages, you'll learn how to self-assess your work posture and adjust your workstation setup to fit your personal preferences so you can work more comfortably, safely, and efficiently.

How to Sit with a Neutral Posture

In ergonomics, you're looking for the sweet spot that you want to obtain in your workspace, and every posture you're in is a neutral or optimal posture for you.

Neutral postures are the ideal body positions that will allow you to become more comfortable and remain pain-free in the office workspace. When you work in neutral postures, you reduce the stress on your muscles and joints, which decreases your risk of getting injured.

It's all about improving your setup without buying expensive pieces of equipment.

Without working in neutral postures, there's no way that you will ever be able to work pain-free. By adjusting the workstation setup to optimally position your devices (including your chair), you can finally work pain-free and make a tremendous improvement in the quality of your life.

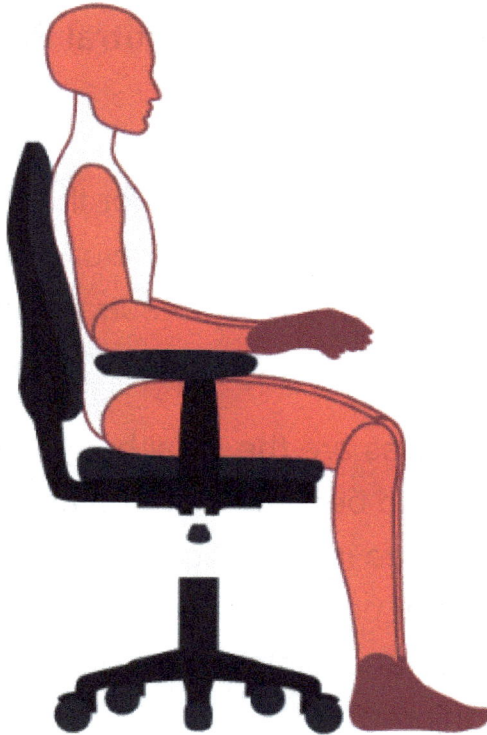

To achieve a neutral posture, remember these
seven things.

1. Your ears are in line with your shoulders.
2. Your head, neck, and trunk are facing
   forward.
3. Your shoulders are relaxed and pulled slightly
   back.
4. Your elbows are close to your body and bent
   at a 90-degree angle.

5. Your back is flush against the chair's back, and the S curve of your lower back is supported.
6. Your thighs are parallel to the floor, and your knees are level or slightly lower than the hips, and there's NO pressure to the back of your knees.
7. Your feet are flat and resting comfortably on the floor or on a footrest.

Home Office Ergonomics

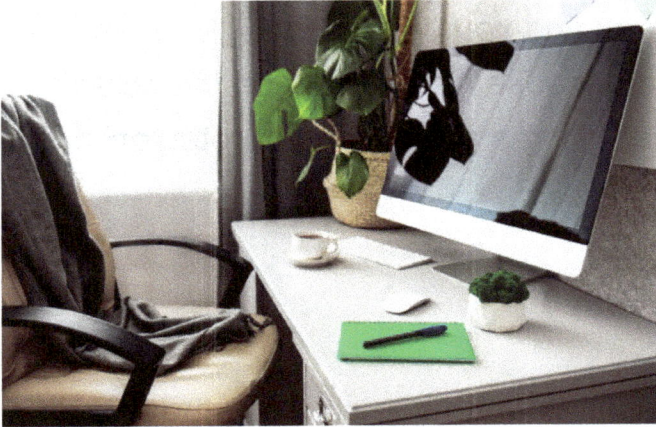

There are five essential elements of your home office setup, and they include your chair, monitor, keyboard, mouse, and how you organize your computer workstation.

Dedicated Workspace

Now, when you're setting up your home office, your primary goal should be to find a dedicated workspace for keying, mousing, and writing.

Try decluttering your work surface, and keep surge protectors and wires organized and tucked away to prevent tripping over them. You want to ensure you have sufficient lighting, preferably natural light, and set your monitor perpendicular to the window to avoid glare.

And if you find yourself squinting a lot and leaning forward because it's hard to see the screen, consider using a glare screen protector[2] or blackout blinds.[3]

Get Creative

Now, given your unique situation, having a dedicated and reliable workstation might not be feasible. So wherever you choose to set up, you'll probably have to get creative to make your physical workspace support your body in a neutral posture.

If you find yourself getting stressed by external noise and it's affecting your focus, try using a headset or noise-canceling headphones.[4]

---

[2] Search online or at a reputable store for antiglare screen protector or matte screen protector.
[3] Search online or at a reputable store for blackout window roller blinds, blackout window shades for room darkening, blackout blinds, or portable blackout curtain.
[4] Search online or at a reputable store for wired/wireless headsets or noise cancelling headphones.

Your Chair

Comfort and good posture are vital in being more productive at work, even if you're working from home.

Avoid the Couch, Bed, or Exercise Ball

You want to avoid the couch or bed as your makeshift workspace, even if it feels cozy. They can lead to slouched postures and put too much pressure on your spine and wreak havoc on your back over the long term.

And the same goes for exercise balls. You want to save those for your home gym workouts and not as your permanent office chair, as research has shown that it can encourage slouching and lead to back problems.[5]

---

[5] Diane E. Gregory, Nadine M. Dunk, and Jack P. Callaghan. "Stability Ball Versus Office Chair: Comparison of Muscle Activation and Lumbar Spine Posture during Prolonged Sitting." *Human Factors* Spring 2006 48:1, 142–153. DOI: 10.1518/001872006776412243.

What Makes a Good Ergonomic Chair?

Sitting with slouched posture on a lousy chair can tighten and fatigue your back muscles. And if your low back is unsupported, it can put too much pressure on your spinal discs. That's why having a fully adjustable office chair[6] is recommended to have an ergonomic work environment. There are only **five major office chair adjustments** that you need to make so that your chair fits you perfectly.

First, there are **seven recommended features of an ergonomic chair** that you should look for when assessing the one you're currently using or if you're in the market to purchase a new one.

---

[6] Search online or at a reputable store for ergonomic home office computer desk chairs.

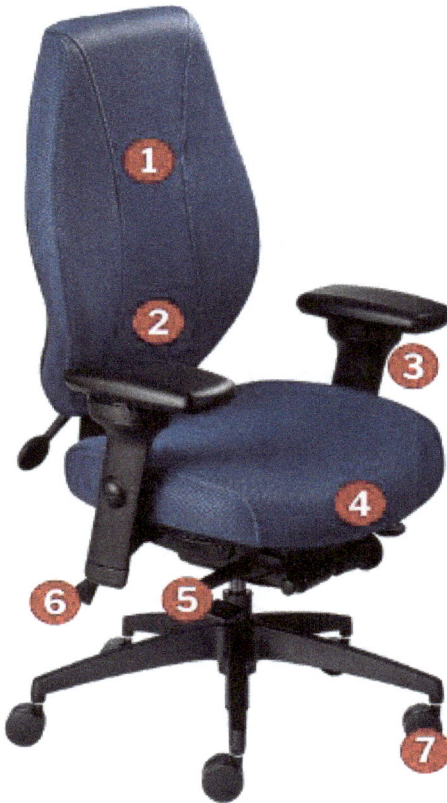

1. Breathable upholstery.
2. Adjustable lumbar support that moves up and down.
3. Adjustable armrests that move up and down and left and right.
4. Seat pan with a rounded waterfall edge.
5. Adjustable seat pan that moves up and down and forward and backward.
6. Tilting mechanism that tilts the chair backward and forward.
7. Five-caster base that rotates the chair 360 degrees.

Five Office Chair Adjustments So It Fits You Perfectly

So now that you know the recommended ergonomic chair features, let's go over the **five essential office chair adjustments**.

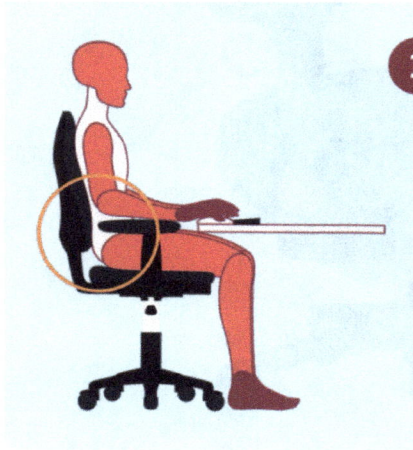

The backrest must support the lower back (lumbar region).

Adjust the lumbar support height to fit into the deepest part of the curve in your lower back.

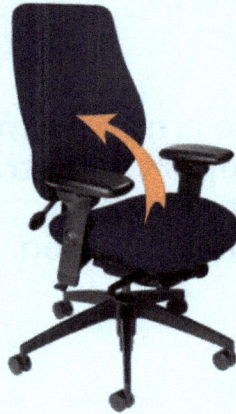

The backrest must tilt backward.

Adjust the tilt of the chair's back so that it's upright and tilted back for your comfort.

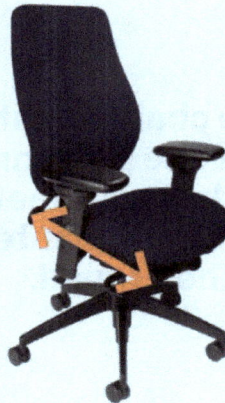

The seat pan must comfortably fit your thigh length.

Adjust the seat pan depth so that there's adequate thigh support, and you can fit two to three fingers between the back of your knees and the front edge of your chair.

The armrests must support a neutral shoulder and elbow position.

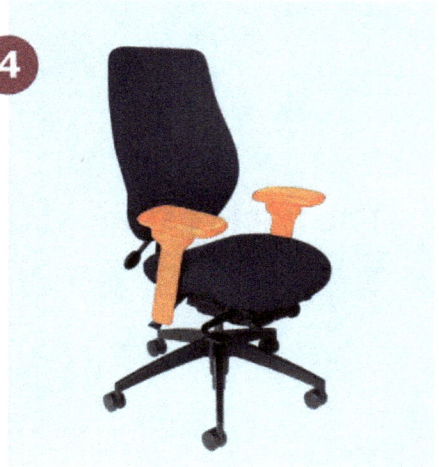

Adjust the armrests, so they're slightly below your elbows when your shoulders are relaxed.

The chair height must be positioned so that your feet are firmly planted on the ground.

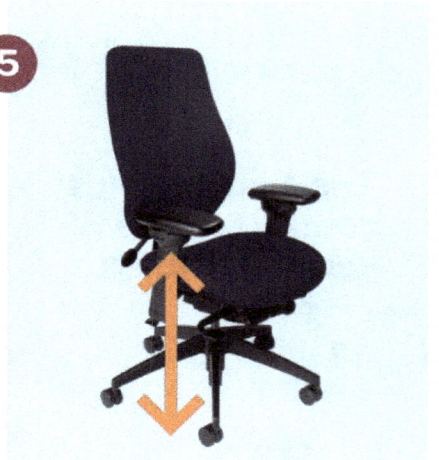

Adjust the seat pan height so that your feet rest flat on the floor and your knees are slightly lower than your hips.

Break Strategy

Even with the most ergonomic setup, risks can still be present, especially without appropriate work breaks. Research has consistently highlighted the strong link between prolonged sitting and back pain.

Over time, this can contribute to lost productivity and the costs associated with workers' compensation claims. That said, choosing an effective break strategy shouldn't be overlooked.

To improve your overall health, wellness, and productivity at work, take frequent microbreaks every 20 to 30 minutes for about 1 to 2 minutes.

During those breaks, incorporate full-body postural changes, such as moving from a seated workstation to standing or taking a quick walk, or if you're already standing or using a sit-stand workstation,[7] transition to sitting or take a brisk walk.

---

[7] Search online or at a reputable store for standing desk, height-adjustable desk, stand-up desk, or standing workstation.

Your Monitor

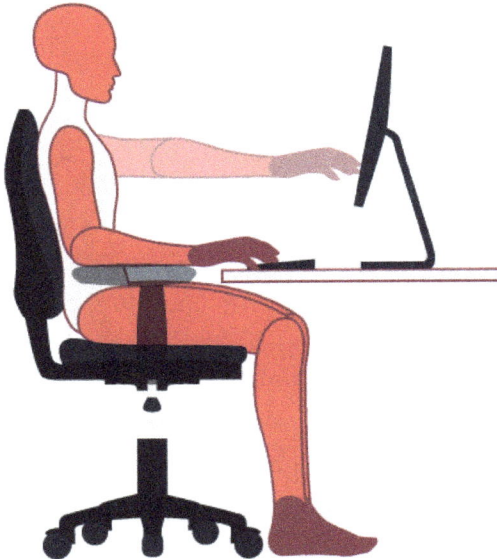

When it comes to computer monitor ergonomics, the two factors to consider are height and distance. You want to position your monitor directly in front of you about an arm's length away and adjust the height so that the top line of print is slightly lower than your eye level. If you wear bifocals, trifocals, or progressive lenses, then you should set the monitor even lower.

How Do You Know Your Monitor Is in an Optimal Position?

When you have a non-neutral posture, your chin is tilted upward, downward, or to the side. This can lead to neck tightness, pain, or headaches.

Monitor Too High?

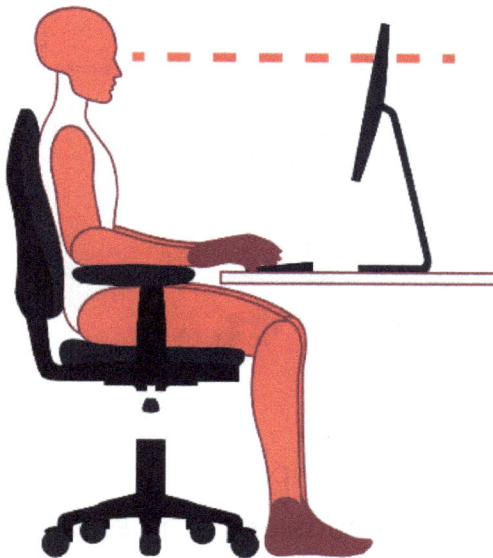

If your monitor is set too high, you'll need to tilt your head back to look up at it. Over time, neck, shoulder, and upper back pain might result. You might also experience dry eyes because there's a tendency to blink less when you're looking up.

If this is the case, lower the monitor or remove the riser from beneath the monitor until the top line of print is at or slightly below eye level, or raise your chair until your eyes are slightly above the top line of print.

Monitor Too Low or Too Far Away?

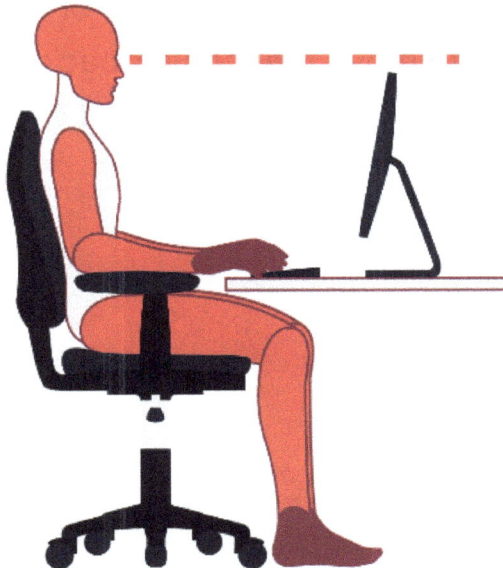

When the monitor is set too low and you find yourself tilting your head down to scan the screen from top to bottom, then raise the monitor until the top line of print is at or slightly below your eye level or even lower if you wear bifocals, trifocals, or progressive lenses.

If you have difficulty reading the screen and need to lean forward, the monitor is too far away. In this case, you want to move the monitor closer until you can sit back and comfortably read the screen without symptoms.

In the reverse case, if your monitor is too close, you can get eye fatigue, blurred vision, or headaches, so you want to move the monitor back until you can comfortably read the screen without experiencing symptoms.

Glare on the Screen

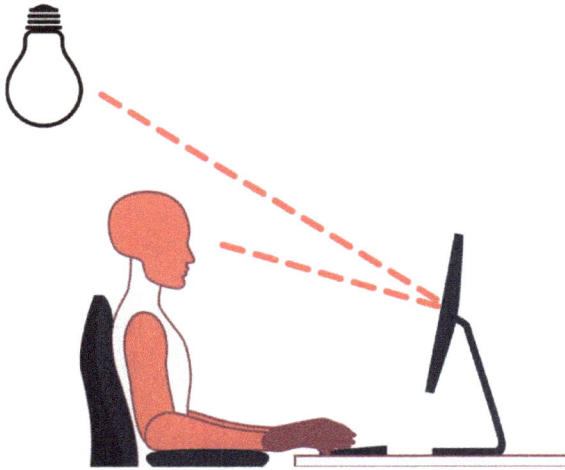

If you see glare on your screen from a task light or overhead lighting, turn the monitor down slightly, dim the task or overhead lights, and draw the blinds or window curtains.

If the glare is coming from the windows, reposition the monitor to perpendicular to the light source.

Multiple Monitors

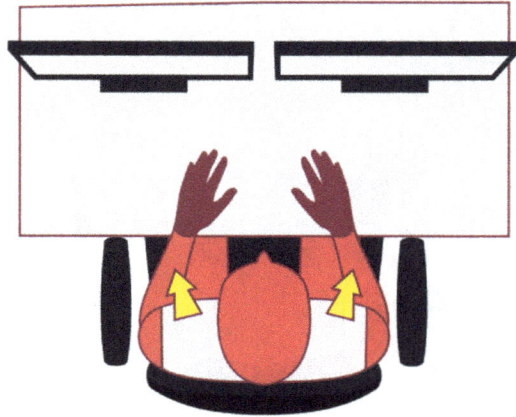

If you're using multiple monitors, position the primary monitor directly in front of you and the other monitors at a 30-degree angle off to the side so you can still view them comfortably without needing to rotate your head.

If you're using both monitors equally, then position them angled in a semicircle. But keep in mind that the tops of the monitors should also be at the same height.

Work from Home Laptop Setup

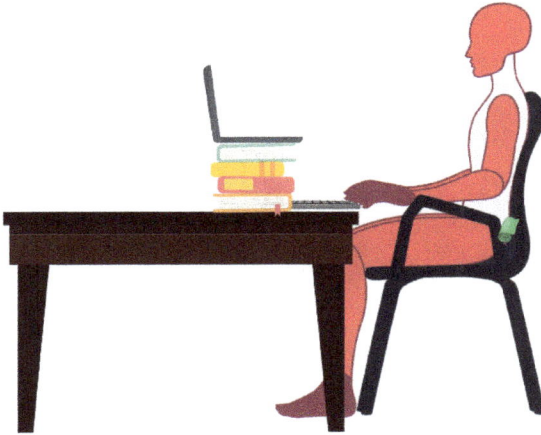

When working from home, chair and desk heights are often mismatched, which makes it challenging to keep your elbows close to the body. If you don't have an adjustable chair, you need to get creative.

A straightforward solution is to elevate your seat with pillows, support your low back with a rolled-up towel or lumbar pad, and then raise your laptop on books. This way, your laptop monitor is closer to eye level.

In this scenario, you'll need an external keyboard and mouse.[8] If your feet aren't resting flat on the floor, use a footstool.

---

[8] Search online or at a reputable store for split keyboard with separate number pad or an ergonomic split keyboard.

Your Keyboard

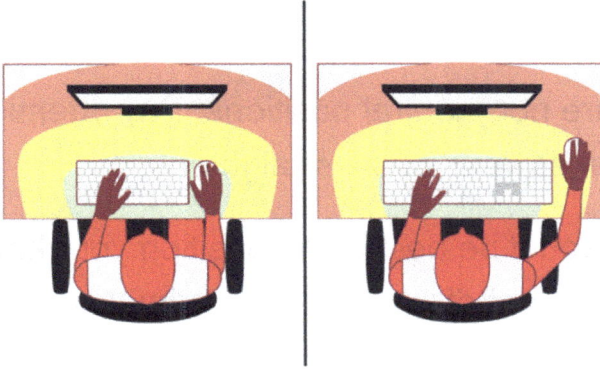

You know that your keyboard is positioned at the correct working height when the following occur.

- Your elbows are close to a body at a 90-degree angle.
- The tops of the home row keys are approximately the same height as your elbows.
- Your wrists are straight and not bent, and your hands are directly lined up with your forearms.

When your keyboard is in a non-neutral position, you might experience pain in your wrists, forearms, elbows, shoulders, and upper back muscles.

Many keyboards have foldable legs under them. Sometimes it helps to flatten the legs or to leave the keyboard at an angle. When the keyboard's back legs are extended, it creates a positive tilt, which causes your wrist to bend upward and create contact stress with the work surface.

These are non-neutral positions. Pay attention to what makes your wrists straighter.

Also, it would be best if you position your keyboard directly in front of you and your primary monitor.

Many people working from home can find themselves working from a nonadjustable table higher than their neutral elbow height.

A work surface that's too high leads to nonoptimal positioning regarding keyboard and mouse ergonomics.

An affordable solution is to purchase a clamp-on keyboard tray[9] and mount it beneath your desk. You

---

[9] Search online or at a reputable store for keyboard tray under desk pull out clamp mount system.

can find various height-adjustable options[10] allowing you to raise, lower, and tilt the keyboard.

It's recommended that the keyboard platform be flat or tilted downward with a negative tilt. It's not recommended to have the keyboard tilt upward, called a positive tilt, as this forces you to bend your wrists back, which can lead to carpal tunnel problems over time.

Split Keyboards

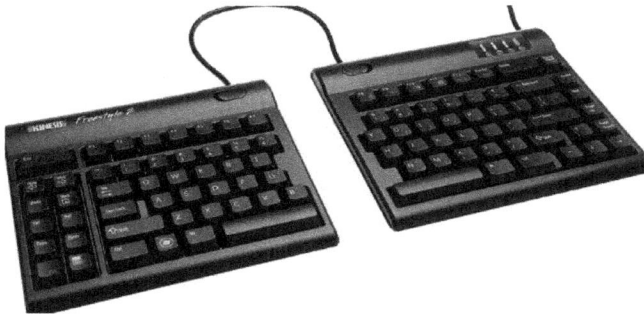

Split keyboards[11] are a good option for individuals with broader shoulders, as they can help prevent wrist deviation.

---

[10] Search online or at a reputable store for keyboard tray with adjustable height platform.
[11] Search online or at a reputable store for split design ergonomic keyboard.

If you don't use a 10-key number pad (usually located on the right side of a regular keyboard, then a narrower keyboard might be a better fit for you, or one with a detachable number pad, as that can provide more room for your mouse.

Your Mouse

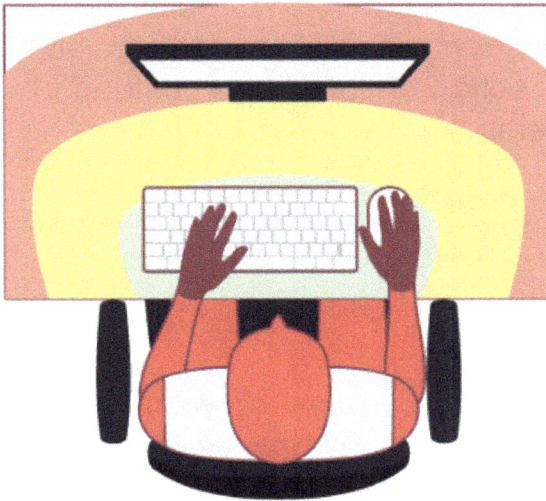

Moving on to mouse ergonomics, let's take a look at your mouse location. When using it, you want to keep your mouse close to your keyboard and use comfortable positions that promote a flat neutral wrist.

Try this technique when using your mouse.

- Gently drop your arm and hand as one unit onto the mouse with your upper arm hanging freely from your shoulder.
- Then center your palm over the mouse and let your fingertips hang over the front and sides.
- When moving the mouse, use your shoulder muscles to generate the force and not your arm by making small circular motions.
- And when clicking the mouse, use the midsection of your finger instead of your fingertip.

Mousing Arm

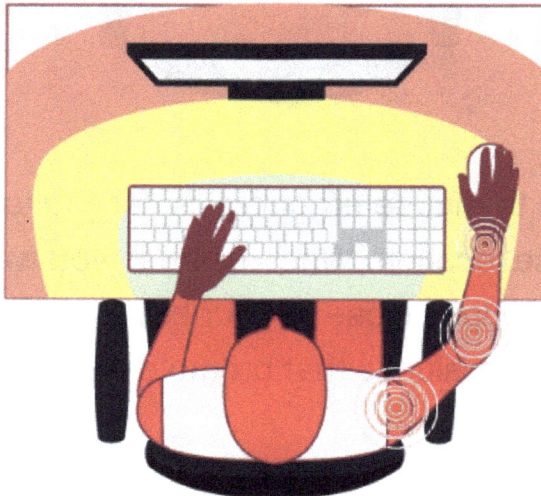

Significant pain symptoms are related to the mouse or in the mousing arm and can range from wrist, elbow, forearm, and shoulder pain.

The major difference between keyboard and mouse pain symptoms...

...is that pain related to non-neutral mouse postures only occurs in one arm, and that is the mousing arm.

More than 90 percent of right arm and shoulder pain is related to the outward positioning of the mouse relative to the right shoulder.

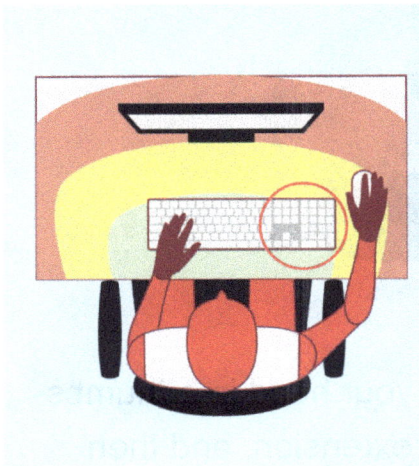

The length of a conventional keyboard is too long for most of us.

The length of a conventional keyboard, which comes with a number pad on the right is too long for most people, so they end up mousing with an outstretched reach far to the right of a neutral position.

So you might want to consider getting a narrower keyboard or one with a detachable number pad, if you're finding that you don't have much use for it.

Numbness or Tingling in Your Hand?

If you're experiencing numbness or tingling in your hand, you might want to look into getting a vertical mouse.[12]

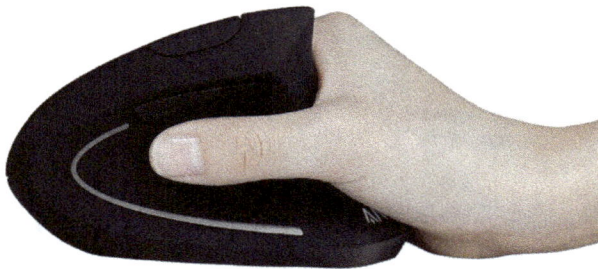

A vertical mouse will keep your hand in a thumbs-up posture, minimize wrist extension, and then reduce the pressure on your carpal tunnel.

---

[12] Search online or at a reputable store for wireless vertical ergonomic optical mouse.

Another solution is to try switching to the other hand for a while to give your uncomfortable hand a rest.

If you change hands, don't forget to change the mouse settings in your computer's control panel.

RollerMouse

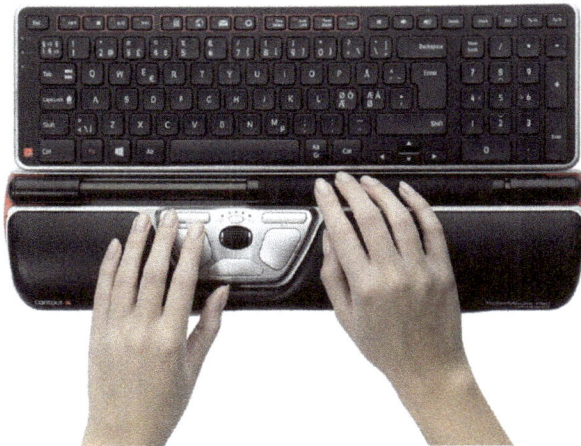

Depending on the job tasks you need to complete, you might find a completely different mouse style that works better for you. So maybe a RollerMouse[13] would be a better fit, as it promotes a

---

[13] Search online or at a reputable store for contour design RollerMouse or ergonomic mouse.

more neutral wrist posture, and you won't ever need to move away from the keyboard.

Workstation Organization

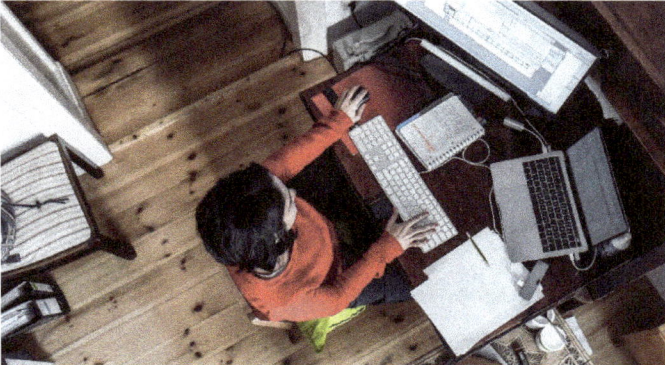

When it comes to working safely, you want to organize your workspace, so there's no need to overreach in any direction. All tasks that you continuously do from your elbows to your fingertips, like using your keyboard and mouse, should be done in what's called your primary work zone.

Your secondary zone is reserved for things you occasionally reach for at about an arm's length away, like a headset or a notepad. And then all things that you seldomly use during your workday should be placed farthest away from you. Also, you might want to consider distributing items on both your right and left sides so that you don't end up overusing one arm more than the other.

Document Holders

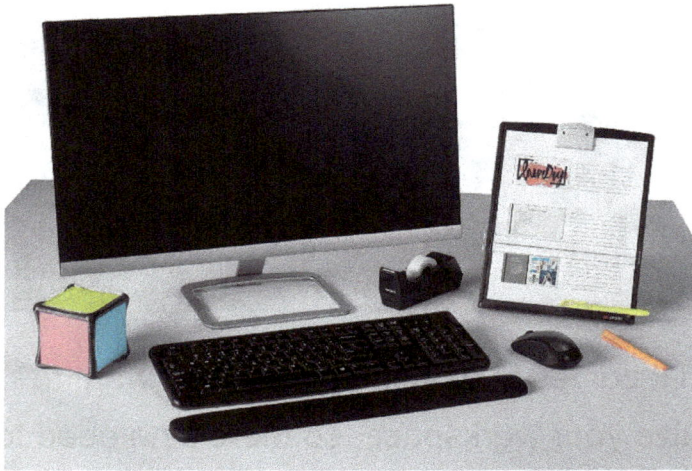

The last thing I'll mention in terms of your home office setup is document holders.[14] This could be helpful if you transcribe documents. It helps prevent neck strains from you repeatedly looking down at your desk and then up at your computer.

You want to position your document holder so that it's in your line of sight. A good location is next to the monitor or between the monitor and the

---

[14] Search online or at a reputable store for document holder, copy holder, or standing clipboard.

keyboard. This way, you can shift your view between the document and the monitor by moving only your eyes and not your head.

Microbreaks

Working remotely from home has many advantages, like cutting your commute time by 100 percent, saving money on gas, fewer distractions, and rocking cozy pajamas in the daytime.

However, sedentary lifestyles and physical inactivity can leave you feeling sluggish and make it hard to concentrate and focus. It can also lead to adverse health outcomes, like cardiovascular disease, cancer, and diabetes.

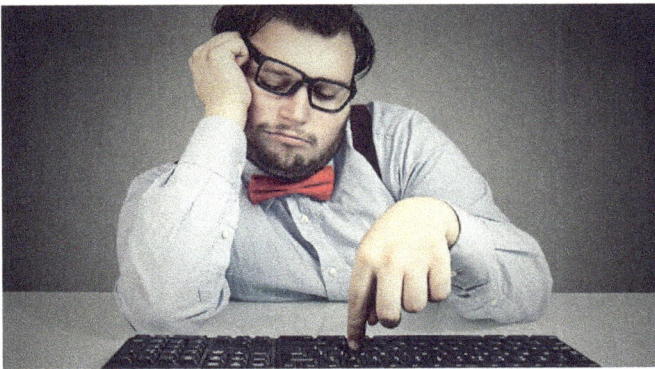

The less you move, the less nutrient-rich oxygenated blood can circulate through your body. This prevents muscles from restoring themselves.

That said, it's essential to break up your workday by inserting microbreaks to prevent fatigue. Breaks also help to keep you from squinting, slouching, and hunching.

The three ergonomic microbreaks are vision, posture, and mental.

Vision Ergonomics

The first microbreak has to do with vision ergonomics. If you're experiencing eyestrain or headaches, then it's an excellent time to take a microbreak and apply the 20-20-20 rule.[15] Every 20 minutes, you want to shift your eyes to look at something 20 feet away for about 20 seconds. This helps give your eyes a rest and prevents eyestrain.

Using the 20-20-20 rule allows your eyes to recalibrate, especially when looking at a screen. You tend not to blink a lot when staring at screens, which can strain the eyes and cause you to lean closer to the monitor, leading to a forward head posture and rounded shoulders.

---

[15] Ashley Marcin, "How Does the 20-20-20 Rule Prevent Eye Strain?" *Healthline* February 3, 2017. https://www.healthline.com/health/eye-health/20-20-20-rule.

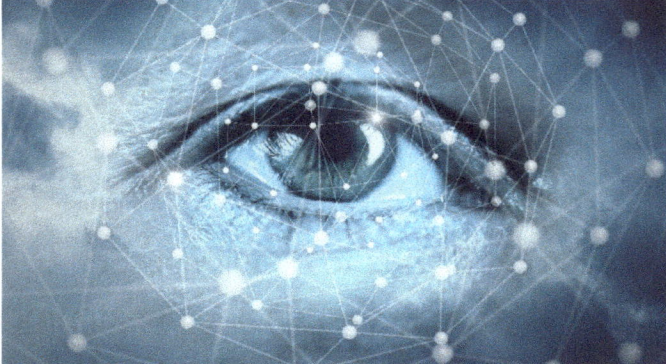

Visual Clarity

For better visual clarity, follow these **five tips.**

1. Adjust your monitor screen brightness, contrast, and font size to make your eyes comfortable looking at the screen.
2. Use the palming technique, where you lightly press your palms over your eyes for about 20 seconds.
3. Clean your monitor screen at least once a week.
4. Blink more often to keep your eyes well lubricated, or use artificial tears.
5. Get your eyes checked annually.

Posture Ergonomics

Microbreak number two is posture ergonomics. The more frequently you change your posture, the less tired you feel by the end of the workday. So it's good to take microbreaks from repetitive tasks or static postures every half hour or so for a few minutes before resuming that activity or posture. A Cornell University study recommends 20-8-2.[16] The way this plays out is that in a 30-minute session, you would sit for 20 minutes, stand for 8 minutes, and then move for 2 minutes.

If you calculate that over an eight-hour workday, that's roughly 16 times you're going from sitting to standing. Now, using a sit-stand workstation allows you to go from a seated to a standing position, decreasing muscle fatigue and taking the pressure off your lower back.

---

[16] "Sitting and Standing at Work." Cornell University Ergonomics Web. https://ergo.human.cornell.edu/CUESitStand.html.

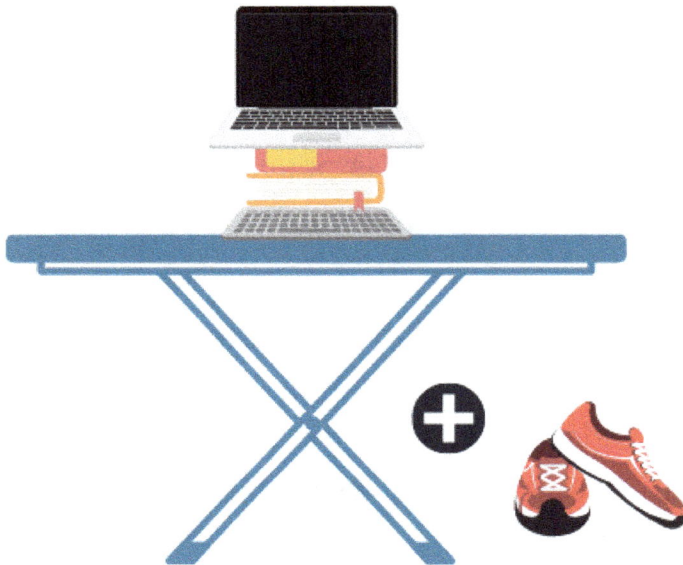

A cost-effective solution for standing desks is to be resourceful with what you already have around the house. So pull out that folded-up ironing board from the closet or use a stack of toilet paper, and you're golden.

Now, remember these three tips when using a standing desk. First, your monitor height should be slightly lower than your eye height and then tilted back about 15 degrees. Second, your desk height should be slightly lower than your elbow height when it's bent approximately 90 degrees. Third, when in a standing position or workspace, you want to stand on something soft or wear running shoes.

Mental Ergonomics

The third microbreak is mental or cognitive ergonomics using the Pomodoro Technique.

After 20 to 25 minutes, take a break. It gives your brain small moments of offline time to reflect and practice mindfulness. Open a tab on your browser and search for "Pomodoro timer." You'll find numerous websites, like https://tomato-timer.com.

***

The common factor that you can take about the three microbreaks is that every 20 minutes or so is a perfect time to change your posture and take a break.

Your Best Posture Is Your Next Posture!

In ergonomics, your best posture is your next posture. So tune into your body. When your fanny says it's been sitting too long, stand. When your feet say they've been standing too long, sit.

Destress at Your Desk

Sedentary lifestyles inevitably result in thousands of hours spent with your body resembling a human question mark, your head jutting forward, rounded shoulders, and your stomach getting closer to your knees.

In this final part of the book, you'll learn several ways you can destress at your desk and improve your posture using breathwork, self-massage, and stretches.

Beat Your Stress with Breath

Monks from Eastern traditions were essentially scientists; they recognized that a wild mind could affect health. So they used meditation techniques to relieve stress so they could stay in balance throughout the day.

Whenever you start to feel irritated or stressed, you can use vagal tone breathing to help you boost the relaxation response of your parasympathetic nervous system to calm you down.[17]

To do it, you want to take slow, relaxed, full breaths, in through your nose for four seconds and then exhale through your mouth for eight seconds.

Shrug your shoulders in sync with your breath. Move your shoulders up with the inhale, and on the exhale, roll them back and down, squeezing your shoulder blades together.

As you breathe, it's ok if your mind starts to wander, and you stop focusing on the breath, just become aware of it, and then come back to the breath and focus on it again. This is the essence of mindfulness—attention to awareness with acceptance.

Practice this vagal tone breathing exercise three times. Remember to take slow, relaxed, full breaths, in through your nose for four seconds and then exhale through your mouth for eight seconds.

---

[17] Roderik J. S. Gerritsen and Guido P. H. Band. "Breath of Life: The Respiratory Vagal Stimulation Model of Contemplative Activity." *Frontiers in Human Neuroscience* 2018. DOI: 10.3389/fnhum.2018.00397.

***

Now, you're going to learn four self-massage techniques and five stretches.

Massage Technique #1: Rake and Twist

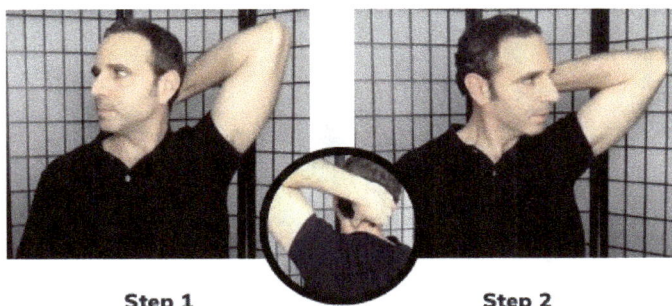

Step 1   Step 2

Step 1: Place your left hand on the back of your neck. Turn your head to the right. Underneath the tips of your fingers are the suboccipitals.

Step 2: Take a deep breath in and exhale as you tighten and rake (drag) your fingers across the back of your neck while you turn your head to the left (toward your elbow).

Maintain tension in your fingertips as you perform the rake move. Move down the back of your neck and stop when you reach the shoulders.

Repeat this rake-and-twist technique three times or until you feel a loosening of the posterior neck musculature. Repeat on the other side of the neck, using the right hand on the left side of your neck.

75

Massage Technique #2: Lobster Claw

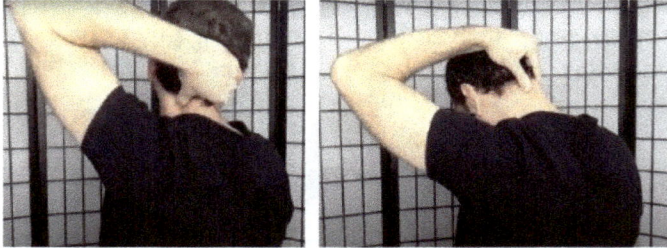

Step 1   Step 2

Step 1: Look up and grasp the back of your neck using your hand like a lobster pincer.

Step 2: Take a deep breath in and exhale as you pull the muscle tissue away as you look down, pinching your fingers together like a lobster claw.

As you nod your head down, try to bring your chin to your chest.

Repeat several times and then switch sides.

Massage Technique #3: Pinch, Lift, and Lateral Flex

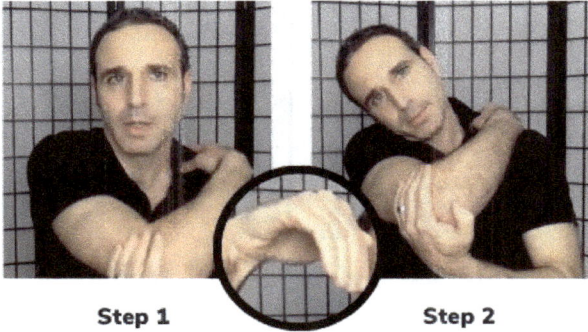

Step 1   Step 2

Step 1: Grip your upper trapezius muscle (across the top of your shoulder) with the fingers of your opposite hand. Cradle your elbow with your palm to support it. Squeeze the trap and lift the muscle tissue a bit.

Step 2: Take a deep breath in and exhale as you laterally flex your neck, bringing your ear toward your shoulder for a few seconds, stretching that muscle tissue. Rotate your head. Repeat several times and then switch sides.

Alternatively, if it's too challenging to pinch the muscle, you can use the fingertips (see middle image) to pin down any knots and laterally flex your neck to the opposite shoulder.

Massage Technique #4: Hook and Knead

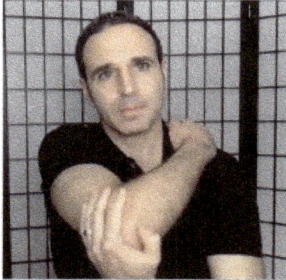 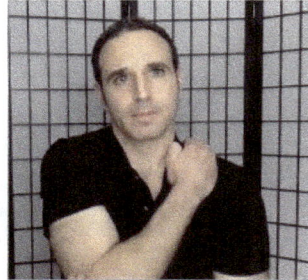

Step 1   Step 2

Step 1: Hook your fingertips on any tight knots you can feel on your upper trapezius muscle.

Step 2: Dig your fingertips down and drag them forward and then release; pulling down on your elbow with the other hand helps control your fingers' movement.

Move laterally from where the top of the shoulder meets the neck to the edge of the shoulders. Switch sides.

***

Now, let's move on to the stretching sequence.

Stretch #1: Chin Tucks

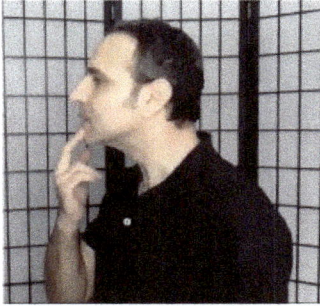 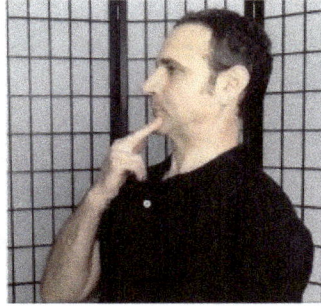

Step 1　　　　　　　　**Step 2**

Chin tucks are good for reversing forward head posture and strengthening the anterior neck muscles. Chin tucks resemble a chicken head's movement as it clucks.

Step 1: Use your index and middle fingers to guide you by placing them on your chin.

Step 2: Retract your neck and hold that position for three to five seconds.

The more of a double chin you create, the better. Repeat five times.

Stretch #2: Lateral Flexion

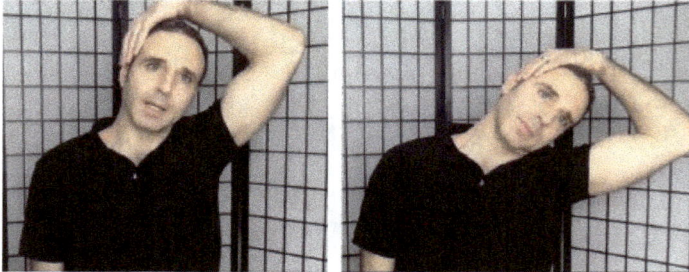

Step 1   Step 2

Step 1: Look straight ahead and begin with Stretch #1 Chin Tuck, so your ears are aligned with your shoulders.

Step 2: Drape your hand over your ear, and pull your head down toward your shoulder.

Hold for a few seconds and then release.

Repeat ten times and then repeat on the opposite side.

Stretch #3: Shoulder Squeeze with Neck Extension

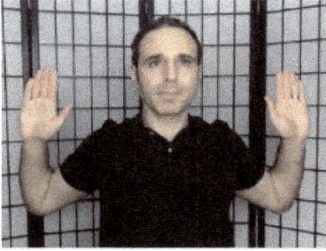 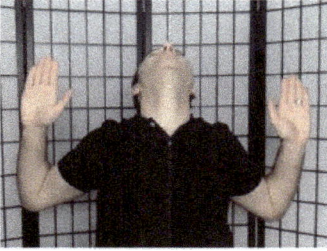

Step 1   Step 2

Step 1: Inhale and then squeeze your shoulder blades together, forming the letter W with your arms.

Step 2: Extend your neck back by raising your chin, tilting your head backward, and looking up.

You want to hold these two movements for about three to five seconds, and then you will exhale and do Stretch #4, Forward Curl with Interlaced Fingers.

Stretch #4: Forward Curl with Interlaced Fingers

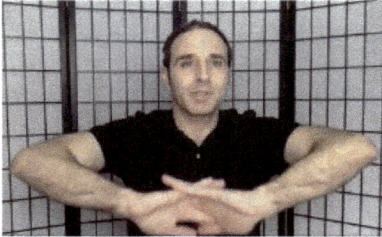 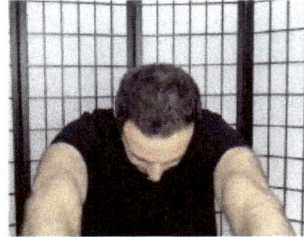

Step 1   **Step 2**

This exercise continues the last movement, so remember to exhale out through your mouth as you do it.

Step 1: Interlace your fingers so that your palms are facing away from you.

Step 2: Extend your arms in front of you as you perform a forward curl, rounding your back and flexing your neck, so your chin touches your chest.

Stretch for four to eight seconds. Repeat three to five times.

Stretch #5: Seated Side Bend

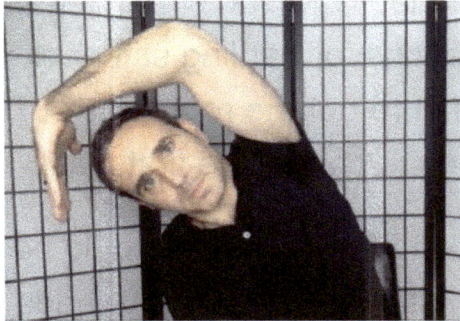

Step 1: Begin by placing your right palm on your left knee.

Step 2: Inhale, and as you exhale, reach your left hand over your head with your palm facing down. You should feel a stretch on the side of your torso.

Final Thoughts

Even though massage and stretching are my go-to recommendations for battling stiff necks, it's essential to figure out the root cause of why you're feeling your neck pain in the first place.

If you're working from home, it could be that you're constantly twisting and tilting your head down to look at the paperwork on your desk and then back up at the monitor. Or maybe it's because your monitor is too far away, and you need to strain your neck forward to see the screen.

Whatever it might be, I want to invite you to take my free self-assessment quiz to determine how much you know about setting up an ergonomic home office.

Access the quiz at https://fitergonomics.com/quiz.

Troubleshooting Pain Working from Home

Since the COVID-19 pandemic, working from home has become the new standard.[18] Some companies like Google, Twitter, and Shopify have offered their employees work-from-home stipends to purchase ergonomic equipment.

However, numerous companies with limited budgets cannot supply all their staff with identical workstation setups at home like back at the office.

This leaves many remote workers to set up their makeshift workstations at their dining room tables, kitchen counters, or even children's playrooms.

Work-from-home injuries are more common than ever with the abundance of remote workers. Haphazardly setting up your home office without understanding basic ergonomic principles can result

---

[18] Emily Courtney. "Remote Work Statistics: Navigating the New Normal." *Flexjobs.* https://www.flexjobs.com/blog/post/remote-work-statistics/.

in neck strains, back spasms, and repetitive stress injuries, such as carpal tunnel and tennis elbow.

Stiff Neck and Headaches

Awkward postures are all too common when using a laptop due to its several ergonomic design flaws like the following.

- The inability to position both the monitor and the keyboard/mouse at the correct height.
- Overuse of index finger from mousing.
- The smaller screen size can encourage forward head posture to view the monitor.

Long-term laptop use can contribute to forward head postures as you need to crane your neck to see the screen. Maintaining forward head postures to look down at your laptop screen is hard to avoid.

If done for prolonged periods, it can strain your neck muscles, cause headaches, and place unnecessary pressure on your cervical spinal discs.

Preventing neck cricks while at your computer comes down to sitting correctly in your chair. When deeply engaged during screen time, you forget that you've evolved into a human and succumb to the caveman or cavewoman slouch.

Every inch the head moves away from the midline, that's an added 10 pounds of pressure on the neck.

When the neck flexes forward just four inches, it can result in 40 pounds of force. That sustained pulling on the posterior neck muscles at their attachment points can conceivably cause a 40-pound headache in the forehead and around the eyes' orbit.

Now, this makes a case for doing chin tucks and maintaining a more neutral neck posture, right?

Take microbreaks every 25 minutes using the Pomodoro Technique.[19] Get up for a short stretch break or a trip to get a drink to prevent physical and mental fatigue.

When your monitor is too high, you can strain your neck when tilting your head to look up at it. To remedy this, adjust your monitor's screen height to be slightly below eye level or even lower if you're wearing bifocals, trifocals, or progressive lenses.

Use a three-ring binder to raise it closer to eye level, or get a laptop stand[20] if you're working with a laptop.

---

[19] Use the Tomato Timer at https://tomato-timer.com.
[20] Search online or at a reputable store for laptop stand, ergonomic laptop stand, computer stand, or height adjustable laptop riser holder.

Going that route, you'll need a wireless keyboard and mouse to prevent you from looking like a zombie. This revised setup might take a little getting used to, so be mindful of your posture.

Recommended Reading

If You Have Neck and Shoulder Pain from Sitting at Computer—Do These 11 Moves!

https://fitergonomics.com/neck-and-shoulder-pain-from-sitting-at-computer/

***

Upper Back Stiffness

Hunching your back like a gargoyle perched over your keyboard can cause rounded shoulders. Your upper back discomfort might result from resting your elbows on armrests that are too high.

If your armrests don't adjust, they can interfere with keying and mousing, which causes you to overreach your arms.

Who knows...that might also be the culprit that's giving you a boulder-size knot between your shoulder blades.[21]

Finding an ergonomic chair with adjustable armrests that allows you to adjust the armrests' height, width, and pivot is a better option for optimal function and safety.

When sitting at your desk, measure your desk height compared to your elbow height when your elbow is bent 90 degrees and close to your side.

---

[21] "Seven Effective Ways to Get Rid of Deep Knots in Shoulder Blades." *Morgan Massage.* 2021. https://morganmassage.com/2018/11/26/deep-knots-in-shoulder-blades/.

If your elbow height is at or lower than your desk, then your chair height is too low. In this scenario, what typically happens is a person will compensate by either sitting on the edge of the chair or pushing the keyboard/mouse farther away from the desk.

Always keep your elbow height higher than your desk height.

By troubleshooting your discomfort with simple tweaks to your work habits, you can relieve the onset of muscle fatigue and learn how to work more efficiently.

Recommended Resources

Reverse Bad Posture Exercises (Udemy)

https://www.udemy.com/course/reverse-bad-posture-exercises/

***

Low Back Strains

Sitting too long at your desk all day in awkward postures without getting up for a break can put pressure on your low back muscles.

Chairs without sufficient lumbar support can contribute to low back pain. Over time, sedentary work can cause uncomfortable muscle strains that can pave the way for herniated discs and chronic pain conditions.

Most dining room chairs and even high-end lounge chairs aren't adjustable and lack the proper lumbar support you need if a chair is functioning as your office chair.

Many people will sacrifice their back comfort by leaning forward in their chair to recreate a more optimal viewing angle and a more comfortable hand position to type and use their mouse. An unsupported low back and turtle-neck computer posture is sure way to an ergonomic injury.

Rolling up a towel to bolster your low back is one solution. If your feet are dangling, use a footstool or a stack of books for your feet to rest on, which will reduce the stress on your lumbar spine.

These are simple ways to improve your chair comfort; however, now you're faced with the mismatch of your desk height being too high or low, leading to overreaching and contact stress of your forearm pressing into the hard surface of the work surface edge.

Listen to your body—when your fanny says it's been sitting too long, stand, and if your feet say they've been standing too long, sit.

As suggested previously, stick to the 20-8-2 rule. Every 20 minutes, get up from sitting, stand for 8 minutes, and then do 2 minutes of moving, like going to the bathroom or getting a snack. You might also want to consider using a standing desk converter, so transitioning from a sitting to an upright posture is more fluid.

Recommended Reading

Nine Back Injury Prevention Exercises to Do While Working from Home

https://fitergonomics.com/back-injury-prevention-exercises/

***

Carpal Tunnel and Tennis Elbow

Another common mishap when working at a work surface that is too high while seated on a too low chair is contact stress and overreaching.

What happens next is your forearms have to stretch forward to reach the keyboard, and your elbows fall out of that neutral posture (being close to your sides).

Continuous pressure against (leaning on) the wrist rest, a hard work surface edge, or armrests with the wrists, forearms, or elbows can lead to inflammatory and disabling repetitive stress injuries, such as carpal tunnel and lateral epicondylitis (aka tennis elbow).

Numbness in the Elbows, Wrist, Hands, or Fingers?

Excessive typing and overuse of a computer mouse can lead to repetitive strain injuries, also referred to as RSI.

Carpal tunnel syndrome is a common RSI caused when the palm's median nerve is compressed and inflamed. Symptoms range from pain and tingling to weakness in the hands.

Many people have lousy keyboard habits that can irritate the carpal tunnel. One example is typing with awkwardly bent wrists because the keyboard is too high or low.

Keep your elbows bent in an "L" shape and your forearms, wrists, and hands in a straight line.

Gripping, finger clicking, and dragging your computer mouse can lead to muscle soreness in your shoulder, referred to as mouse shoulder.

If this is the case, select an ergonomic mouse that matched your hand's size. When you use a mouse while keying, it is essential to access it without overreaching or using awkward postures. To achieve this, position your mouse as close to the keyboard as possible.

***

When you find yourself dealing with one ergonomic dilemma after another, and it's giving you decision fatigue, that's a sign that it's time to book a remote ergonomic assessment. A professional ergonomist can guide you toward safer solutions so you can avoid getting hurt and be more productive.

See "Home Office Ergonomic Assessment" at https://fitergonomics.com/home-office-ergonomic-assessment/.

Recommended Reading

This 10-Minute at Home Treatment for Tennis Elbow Pain Really Works

https://fitergonomics.com/at-home-treatment-for-tennis-elbow/

About Morgan Sutherland

Morgan Sutherland has been a massage therapist for over 20 years and a certified ergonomics assessment specialist since 2020. He has numerous self-published books on Amazon about fixing bad posture and getting rid of back pain. In addition, Morgan has created three online courses about cupping, back pain, and posture, and he also runs a health and wellness blog.

Growing up, his father, a documentary filmmaker,[22] suffered from chronic neck and shoulder pain, which Morgan imagined was caused by the countless hours spent sitting twisted like a pretzel in front of the editing machine.

Morgan's father would get tremendous relief from weekly massages, yet he'd always spring back to that pretzel-like posture, and that vicious cycle of pain would continue. Years later, Morgan built a reputation for himself as a massage therapist who

---

[22] See David Sutherland Productions at http://davidsutherland.com/.

specialized in chronic pain. And after working on thousands of clients, he realized that the root cause of their discomfort stemmed, in many cases, from their poor posture and ergonomics.

When the pandemic struck in 2020 and so many people started working from home, Morgan hit the pause button on his massage business and pursued his passion for posture. This led him to become certified as an ergonomics specialist and soon after he launched Fit Ergonomics.

Amazon Website
https://amazon.com/author/morgansutherland

Health and Wellness Blog
https://morganmassage.com/

Fit Ergonomics Website
https://fitergonomics.com/

Other Books by Morgan Sutherland

The Essential Lower Back Pain Exercises Guide: Treat Lower Back Pain at Home in Twenty-One Days

***

Reverse Bad Posture Exercises: Fix Neck, Back and Shoulder Pain in Just 15 Minutes per Day (Reverse Your Pain Book 1)

***

Reverse Pain in Hips and Knees: Super-Effective Back, Hip, and Knee Stretches and Strengthening Exercises (Reverse Your Pain Book 2)

***

Reverse Back and Shoulder Pain: Effective Home Exercises for Back and Shoulder Pain (Reverse Your Pain Book 3)

***

Best Treatment for Sciatica Pain: Relieve Sciatica Symptoms, Piriformis Muscle Pain, and SI Joint Pain in Just 20 Minutes or Less Per Day

***

Twenty-One Yoga Exercises for Lower Back Pain: Stretching Lower Back Pain Away with Yoga

***

Resistance Band Workouts for Bad Posture and Back Pain: Step-by-Step Illustrated Resistance Band Workouts for Back Pain Sufferers

***

DIY Low Back Pain Relief: Nine Way to Fix Low Back Pain So You Can Feel Like Yourself Again

www.ingramcontent.com/pod-product-compliance
Lightning Source LLC
Chambersburg PA
CBHW060248030426
42335CB00014B/1631